LAST HELP: PHAGE THERAPY?

FOR 100 YEARS, A SUCCESSFUL ALTERNATIVE TO CONVENTIONAL ANTIBIOTIC TREATMENTS

PAUL ENDERS

Copyright © Paul Enders
All Rights Reserved.

ISBN 978-1-63886-853-8

This book has been published with all efforts taken to make the material error-free after the consent of the author. However, the author and the publisher do not assume and hereby disclaim any liability to any party for any loss, damage, or disruption caused by errors or omissions, whether such errors or omissions result from negligence, accident, or any other cause.

While every effort has been made to avoid any mistake or omission, this publication is being sold on the condition and understanding that neither the author nor the publishers or printers would be liable in any manner to any person by reason of any mistake or omission in this publication or for any action taken or omitted to be taken or advice rendered or accepted on the basis of this work. For any defect in printing or binding the publishers will be liable only to replace the defective copy by another copy of this work then available.

Contents

Acknowledgements	v
1. Introduction	1
2. History Of Phage Therapy	2
3. When Antibiotics Are Power-less	4
4. Different Types Of Phages	9
5. Practical Applications Of Bacteriophages	13
6. Advantages Of Bacteriophage Preparations	16
7. Pros And Cons Of Bacteriophages	19
8. Uses Of Bacteriophages Or Phage Therapy	21
9. Phage Therapy An Alternative To Antibiotics	28
10. The Resistance Of Microorganisms And Ways To Overcome It	32

Acknowledgements

Introduction

By using this book, you accept this disclaimer in full.

No advice

The book contains information. The information is not advice and should not be treated as such.

No representations or warranties

To the maximum extent permitted by applicable law and subject to section below, we exclude all representations, warranties, undertakings and guarantees relating to the book.

Without prejudice to the generality of the foregoing paragraph, we do not represent, warrant, undertake or guarantee:

- that the information in the book is correct, accurate, complete or non-misleading.

- that the use of the guidance in the book will lead to any particular outcome or result.

Limitations and exclusions of liability

The limitations and exclusions of liability set out in this section and elsewhere in this disclaimer: are subject to section 6 below; and govern all liabilities arising under the disclaimer or in relation to the book, including liabilities arising in contract, in tort (including negligence) and for breach of statutory duty.

We will not be liable to you in respect of any losses arising out of any event or events beyond our reasonable control.

We will not be liable to you in respect of any business losses, including without limitation loss of or damage to profits, income, revenue, use, production, anticipated savings, business, contracts, commercial opportunities or goodwill.

We will not be liable to you in respect of any loss or corruption of any data, database or software.

We will not be liable to you in respect of any special, indirect or consequential loss or damage.

Exceptions

Nothing in this disclaimer shall: limit or exclude our liability for death or personal injury resulting from negligence; limit or exclude our liability for fraud or fraudulent misrepresentation; limit any of our liabilities in any way that is not permitted under applicable law; or exclude any of our liabilities that may not be excluded under applicable law.

Severability

If a section of this disclaimer is determined by any court or other competent authority to be unlawful and/or unenforceable, the other sections of this disclaimer continue in effect.

If any unlawful and/or unenforceable section would be lawful or enforceable if part of it were deleted, that part will be deemed to be deleted, and the rest of the section will continue in effect.

Law and jurisdiction

This disclaimer will be governed by and construed in accordance with Swiss law, and any disputes relating to this disclaimer will be subject to the exclusive jurisdiction of the courts of Switzerland.

CHAPTER ONE

Introduction

We live in a world where all types of living sharing a bond, which can be a direct bond or an indirect bond. This is so true when we think about it seriously. Man lives in constant contact and in complex interaction with an innumerable multitude of microorganisms that are present within our universe. A person cannot live without the bacteria, but also not live with too many of them. Every year, many people die from bacterial diseases such as, 3.9 million people from pneumonia, 1.6 million from diarrhea, 1.6 million from tuberculosis, and so on.

This shows that antibacterial or antibiotic therapy has failed these people. Antibiotics were not enough to fight those pathogenic bacteria. There is no need to use antibiotics, which cannot kill bacteria but can only contribute to its side effects.

Here comes the re-evaluation of the idea of using something extraordinary, which was also from the same age as antibiotics, but has never been used in mainstream practice because of the easy access and use of antibiotics in that era. However, it is different now. Most of the bacteria developed a resistance to antibiotics and, hence, cannot kill or eliminate bacteria. Even though doctors who prescribe antibiotics without any need or people who takes antibiotics for every sneeze they get are to blame, these events, unfortunately, have led to the development of severe resistance to antibiotics by bacteria.

Hence, the only way to help those in need with bacterial diseases is through the use of bacteriophages. Bacteriophage therapy became famous in almost all parts of the world, especially in developed countries.

CHAPTER TWO

History of Phage Therapy

Phage therapy kills pathogenic bacteria and can act as an alternative to antibiotic therapy. The idea of phage therapy was put forward in 1917 by one of the discoverers of Bacteriophages, Canadian scientist F. D'Erell (1873-1949). However, with the advent of penicillin in 1929, which marked the beginning of the era of antibiotics in medicine, phage therapy was pushed into the background.

In 1896, Ernest Hankin said that the water of the Ganges and Yamuna rivers in India had significant antibacterial activity, which persisted after passing through a porcelain filter with pores of very small size but was eliminated by boiling. He particularly studied the effect of an unknown substance on Vibrio cholera and suggested that drinking water from these rivers was responsible for the prevention of the spread of epidemics of cholera. However, he did not later explain this phenomenon.

In 1898, lysis of bacteria (anthrax bacillus) was observed by Russian microbiologist, N.F. Gamaleja, for the first time. In 1915 English scientist, F. Tuort, described the phenomenon of lysis of Staphylococcus in the purulent and open wound and this led to the first "virus that eats bacteria" found in the cultures of a calf lymph. After the discovery, this phenomenon of lysis is described as "Tuort's phenomenon". In 1917, Felix D'Erell made a similar discovery and gave them the name "Bacteriophages", using the suffix "phage". Nevertheless, the work continued with bacteriophages and their role in phage therapy was constantly analyzed. This became a model to study basic biological processes of the group of phages of E. coli. Major scientific breakthrough in phage therapy was seen in the 20th century.

In the 1920s and 1930s, phage therapy was used to treat bacterial infections in the United States. It was widely used for the treatment of the Red Army, to cope with dysentery, and helped the sick soldiers quickly back into operation. However, when antibiotics were produced by the 1950s, antibiotic therapy became a cornerstone in the treatment of many diseases. It put an end to further research and development of phage therapy. Nevertheless, the Soviet Union continued the use of phage therapy and conducted successful research in this field. In Russia and Eastern Europe, such as Germany and Poland, phage therapy has been used successfully against diphtheria, tetanus, gangrene, scarlet fever, and meningococcal. Phage therapy shows great promise in the treatment of many diseases, especially in the bacterial diseases. In our society, the epidemic of resistance to antibiotics and the harmful effects of excessive use of antibiotics are well known. In this regard, phage therapy has obvious advantages compared to antibiotics. In addition, phages remain intact and maintain healthy microflora, preventing excessive intestinal bacterial colonization. Phages are able to fend off opportunistic organisms without any adverse reactions. This feature makes them a valuable tool for promoting the preservation of health.

In the 1980's, the effectiveness of antibiotic treatment significantly decreased, the bacteria had actively developed drug resistance. To create a new potent antibiotic, drug companies today need to spend an average of 10 years and $800 million. This has led to an increased interest in phage therapy. At the beginning of 2000, Glenn Morris and the University of Maryland (USA), in cooperation with the Research Institute of Bacteriophages, Microbiology and Virology in Tbilisi, established the test of phage preparations to obtain a license for their use in the United States. Moreover, in July 2007, bacteriophages were approved for use in the United States. Over the past few years, studies of the properties of bacteriophages have been carried out in Russia, Georgia, Poland, France, Germany, Finland, Canada, USA, UK, Mexico, Israel, India, and Australia.

CHAPTER THREE

When Antibiotics Are Power-Less

Phages, as an intracellular parasite of bacteria, depend on the host cell. For example, virtually every stage of development requires the involvement of bacterial enzymes, special structures, etc. Bacterial mutations can, therefore, be quite easily blocked by the development of the phage, making a host cell genetically resistant to the particular phage. To avoid or at least significantly reduce the likelihood of this, experts make and use phage mixtures, "living" in bacteria, of different strains of the same species (or of different types). In this case, mutants exhibiting resistance to one phage are infected and killed by the other. This substantially reduces the proportion of surviving phage-resistant bacteria and the extended time of use of such therapeutic mixtures in the treatment of a particular patient.

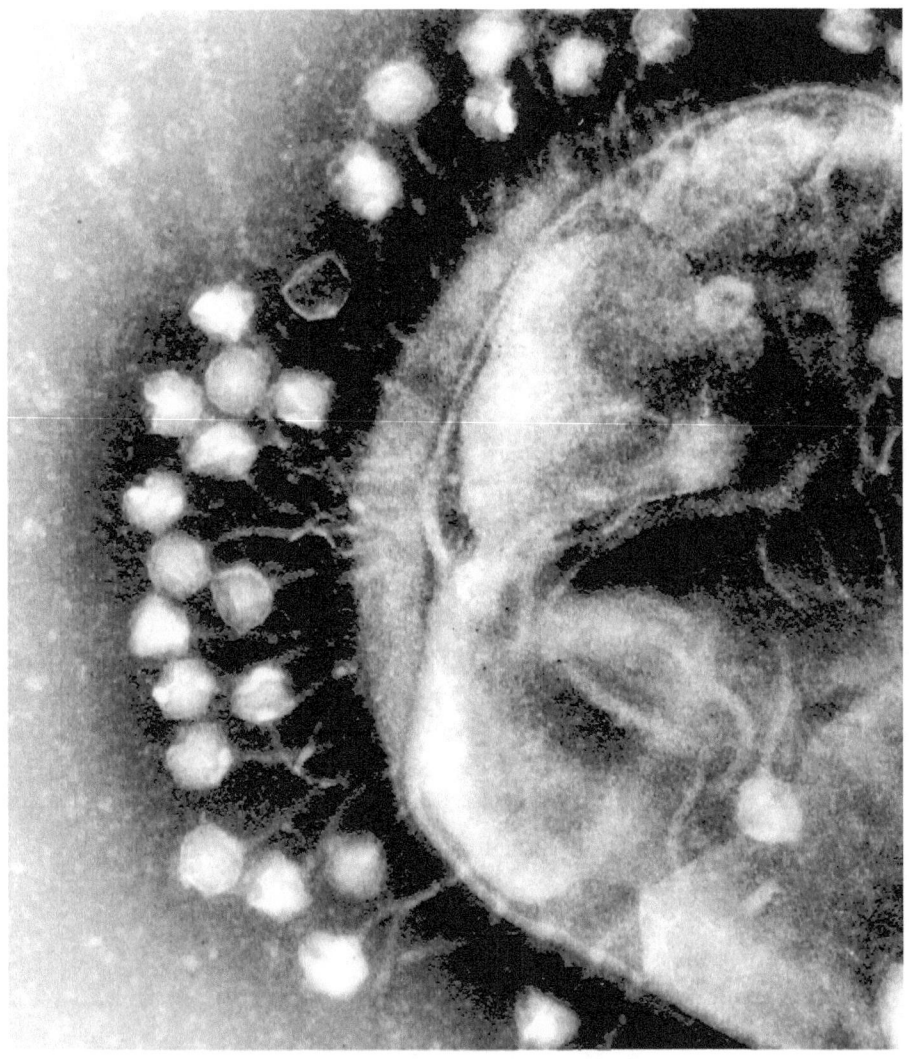

by Dr Graham Beards (en:Image:Phage.jpg) [CC BY-SA 3.0 (http://creativecommons.org/licenses/by-sa/3.0) oder GFDL (http://www.gnu.org/copyleft/fdl.html)], via Wikimedia Commons

The effectiveness of this method of treatment can be assessed by the total number of phage species that are active in different species of bacteria and their conservation. For example, we conducted rapid classification of groups of samples of virulent phages of Pseudomonas Aeruginosa.

Pseudomonas Aeruginosa showed a significant part of them represented by a single phage. It follows that many more species active on these bacteria are not found. On the other hand, individual phages of the same species are found repeatedly. So, not yet identified the species that may be just missing for phage therapy, while introducing into the mixture and let a little different, but closely related phages may be totally meaningless.

Therefore, the search for new types of phages becomes the priority. When these bacteriophages with optimal properties for the treatment choice are found, it will be necessary to establish the natural boundaries for a variety of features that will allow you to create the optimal therapeutic mixture. Generally, in order to maintain high efficiency of the combined phage preparations, we often have to replace some other phages. That is why pharmacies may offer products under the same label, containing completely different sets of bacteriophages. It depends on what source of bacteria strains were used for the selection of these phages.

In addition, sometimes there are paradoxical cases where the drug, according to the attached description, contains at least 10 different specific phages against Escherichia coli and, while confirming proper activity in one region, is completely useless in another situation. However, the use of mixtures in live phage therapy has advantages due to the speed, relative economy and ease of manufacturing. When these phage mixtures are properly and individually selected for each patient, the components in each phage mixture are highly concentrated and the effectiveness of phage therapy. Furthermore, the use of live phages allows introduction into the body in a minimum amount because they can proliferate until they sense bacteria.

Phage morphology

Phages' dimensions are 20 - 200nm. Most phages are in the form of tadpoles. The complex structure of phages consists of a polyhedral head, which is a nucleic acid, neck, and processes. At the end of the process is the basal lamina, with the radiating strands and the tentacle-like structures. These tentacles serve as a means of attachment of the phage to a bacteria shell. The distal process of the bacteriophage contains the enzyme - lysozyme. This enzyme promotes the dissolution of the shell when phages penetrate the bacteria in order to reach the cytoplasm. Many phages processes are surrounded by a cover, which in some types of phages can be absent.

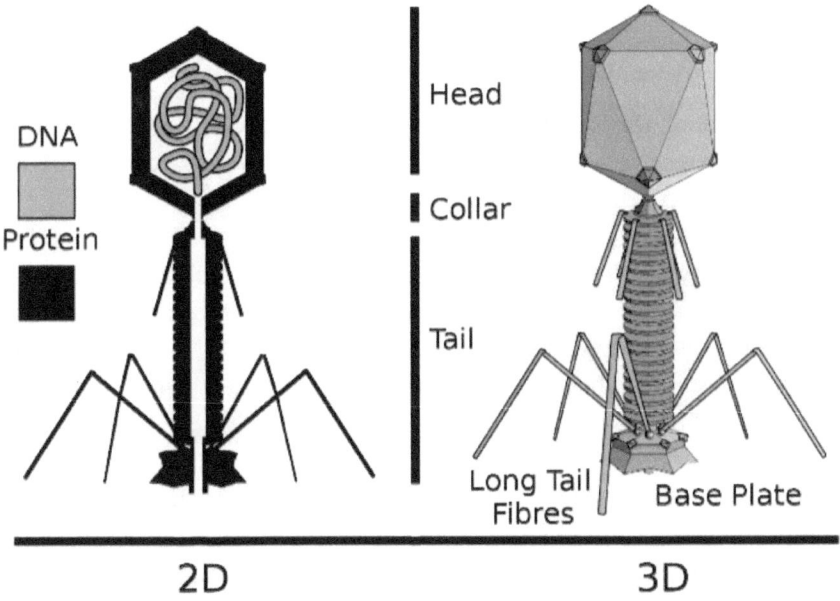

by Adenosine (original); en:User:Pbroks13 (redraw) [CC BY-SA 2.5 (http://creativecommons.org/licenses/by-sa/2.5)], via Wikimedia Commons

There are 5 groups of morphological phages, as follows:

- Bacteriophages with a long process and shrinking cover
- Phages with a long process, but do not possess cover
- Phages with short appendages
- Phages with an analogue process
- The filamentous types of phages

Chemical composition of Phages or Bacteriophages:
Phages are composed of nucleic acids and proteins. Most of them contain 2 sets of DNA in a closed ring. Some phages contain a single strand of DNA or RNA.
According to the specificity of the interaction:

- Polyphagia - interacting with several related species of bacteria.

- Monophagy - phages species - interact with one species of bacteria.
- Typical phages - interact with certain variants of bacteria within a species.

The **action of the standard form of the phage** can be divided into a number of phages. The reaction of phages with bacteria can occur as a productive, non-productive and integrative type.

- Productive type - is formed phage progeny, and the cells are killed.
- When non-productive - cell continues to exist; the interaction process is terminated at an early stage.
- Integrative type - phage genome integrates into the chromosome of the bacteria and coexists with it.

Depending on the type of interaction, phages can be distinguished into **virulent and temperate phages**. Virulent bacteria interact with productive type. Early absorption takes place on the shell of the phage of bacteria due to the interaction of specific receptors. This leads to the penetration or infiltration of viral nucleic acid into the cytoplasm of the bacteria. Under the action of lysozyme, coated bacteria form a small hole in the phage cover and reduced Natural Killer cells are injected. Next, the synthesis of early proteins happens. They provide the synthesis of structural phage proteins, with the replication of phage nucleic acids, and bacterial chromosomes repression activity happens, with the help of early proteins.

Temperate phages interact with either the productive or the integrative type. The productive cycle is similar to virulent type. When integrative cooperation happens, the temperate phage's DNA, after being hit by the cytoplasm, integrates into the chromosome in a certain area. Moreover, during cell division, phages are replicated synchronously with bacterial DNA and these structures are transmitted to daughter cells. This builds the phage DNA - prophage and bacterium containing prophage. This phenomenon is called lysogenicity.

CHAPTER FOUR

Different Types of Phages

Bacteriophage, klebsiella pneumoniae (Klebsiphage), has the ability to specifically kill the bacteria, klebsiella, which causes pneumonia. It is designed for the treatment of septic and enteric diseases caused by bacteria klebsiella-pneumoniae, such as surgical site infections, diseases of the urogenital system, gastrointestinal tract, and chronic inflammatory diseases of the ear, nose, throat, respiratory tract and lungs, generalized septic diseases, and septic neonatal disease.

Bacteriophage, coli (coliphage), has the ability to specifically lyse enteropathogenic E. coli (Escherichia coli), the most important in the etiology of chronic inflammatory diseases. Applied for the treatment and prevention of infections of the skin and internal organs caused by Escherichia coli, such as septic diseases, purulent complications of wounds, burns, abscesses, boils, carbuncles, bursitis, tenosynovitis, osteomyelitis (bone infection), mastitis (infection of mammary gland), pleurisy (affection of pleural membrane), Cholecystitis (gall bladder infection), proctitis (infection or inflammation of rectum) , cystitis (infection of urinary bladder), pyelonephritis (inflammation or infection of kidney pelvis apparatus), endometritis (inflammation of the innermost layer of uterus), vaginitis (inflammation of vagina), salpingo-oophoritis (inflammation of the fallopian tube and ovary), enteritis (inflammation of the large intestine), enterocolitis (inflammation of small intestine and large intestine), and poisoning.

Bacteriophage of coliproteus (Coliproteophage) has the ability to specifically kill common enteropathogenic Escherichia and Proteus (Proteus Mirabilis and Proteus Vulgaris). Applied for the treatment and prevention of enterocolitis, treatment of colpitis, coliproteus etiology and other diseases caused by bacteria coli and proteus, such as cystitis (infection of urinary bladder), pyelonephritis (kidney pelvis infection), endometritis (inflammation of the innermost layer of uterus), salpingo-oophoritis (inflammation of the fallopian tube and ovary), and enteric diseases (diseases of intestine).

Bacteriophage, Pseudomonas aeruginosa, has the ability to specifically kill bacteria pseudomonas aeruginosa. Applied for the treatment and prevention of inflammatory diseases of different organs caused by pseudomonas aeruginosa (diseases of the ear, nose, throat, respiratory tract and lungs, surgical infections, obstetric infections, enteric infections, septic diseases, and chronic inflammatory diseases of the newborn), goitre, as well as prophylactic treatment for postoperative infections and wound infections, and for the prevention of nosocomial infections.

Staphylococcal bacteriophage (Staphylophage) has the ability to lyse staphylococcal bacteria isolated in purulent infections. Applied for the treatment and prophylaxis of purulent infections of the skin, mucous membranes, visceral organs, diseases caused by staphylococcal bacteria, such as sinusitis (inflammation of the sinus), otitis (inflammation of the ear), tonsillitis (inflammation of tonsil), pharyngitis (inflammation of pharynx), laryngitis (inflammation of larynx), tracheitis (inflammation of trachea), bronchitis (inflammation of bronchus), pneumonia (inflammation of lungs), pleurisy (inflammation of pleura), purulent wounds, infected burns, abscess, cellulitis (inflammation of fat tissue), boils, carbuncle, hidradenitis supra (inflammation of sweat glands), mastitis (inflammation of mammary gland), bursitis (inflammation of bursa), osteomyelitis (inflammation of bones), urethritis (inflammation of urethra), cystitis (inflammation of urinary bladder), pyelonephritis (inflammation of kidney pelvis), vaginitis (inflammation of vagina), endometritis (inflammation of innermost layer of uterus), salpingo-oophoritis (inflammation of the fallopian tube and ovary), gastroenterocolitis (inflammation of stomach, small intestine and large intestine), cholecystitis (inflammation of gall bladder), omphalitis (inflammation of umbilicus), sepsis, as well as intestinal dysbacteriosis.

Bacteriophage, streptococcal (Streptophage), has the ability to kill or eliminate streptococcal bacteria isolated in purulent infections. Applied for the treatment and prophylaxis of purulent infections of the skin, mucous membranes, visceral organs, diseases caused by streptococcal, such as sinusitis (inflammation of the sinus), otitis (inflammation of the ear), sore throat, tonsillitis (inflammation of the tonsil), pharyngitis (inflammation of pharynx), laryngitis (inflammation of larynx), tracheitis (inflammation of trachea), bronchitis (inflammation of bronchus), pneumonia (inflammation of lungs), pleurisy (inflammation of pleura), festering wounds, suppurative complications of burns, abscess, cellulitis, boils, carbuncles, hidradenitis supra, mastitis (inflammation of the mammary gland), bursitis, tenosynovitis (inflammation of tendon and synovial membrane), osteomyelitis (inflammation of bones), urethritis (inflammation of urethra), cystitis (inflammation of urinary bladder), pyelonephritis (inflammation of kidney pelvis), vaginitis (inflammation of vagina), endometritis (inflammation of innermost layer of uterus), salpingo-oophoritis (inflammation of fallopian tube and ovary), gastroenterocolitis (inflammation of stomach, small intestine and large intestine), cholecystitis (inflammation of gall bladder), omphalitis (inflammation of umbilicus), pyoderma, sepsis, as well as intestinal dysbacteriosis .

Pyobacteriophage combined form (Pyopoliphage) is able to lyse staphylo-, streptococci, proteus, pseudomonas, and E. coli. It is intended for the prevention and treatment of inflammatory diseases of the ear, nose, throat, sinuses, airways of the lungs, surgical site infections (suppurations, abscesses, cellulitis, osteomyelitis, and peritonitis), urogenital infections (urethritis, cystitis, and pyelonephritis), gynecological infections (vaginitis, endometritis, and salpingo-oophoritis), enteric infections (gastroenterocolitis, cholecystitis, dysbacteriosis) and septic neonatal diseases.

Pyobacteriophage polyvalent form has the ability to specifically lyse staphylo-, streptococci, E. coli, proteus, pseudomonas aeruginosa and klebsiella pneumonia. It is intended for the prevention and treatment of various forms of inflammatory and enteric diseases, such as chronic inflammatory diseases of the ear, nose, throat, respiratory tract, lungs, and pleura; surgical, enteral and urogenital infections; generalized septic diseases, and septic diseases of newborns and infants.

Pyobacteriophage integrated liquid is a mixture of staphylo-, streptococci, enterococci, E. coli, proteus (mirabilis and vulgaris), pseudomonas aeruginosa and klebsiella (pneumonia and oxytoca). Applied for the treatment and prevention of inflammatory and intestinal diseases, such as diseases of the ear, nose, throat, respiratory tract and lungs; surgical, obstetric, and enteric infections; generalized and septic diseases; chronic inflammatory diseases of the newborn, and for the treatment of post-operative wounds.

Therapeutic and prophylactic bacteriophages contain polyclonal virulent bacteriophages with a wide range of activities against bacteria resistant to antibiotics. Phage therapy can be successfully combined with antibiotic therapy.

The idea of using bacteriophages in the treatment of bacterial etiologic diseases should be immediately after their discovery. It still remains one of the most promising ideas, transforming from the opening to the methodology in the field of modern medical nanotechnology. A distinctive feature of bacteriophage therapeutic agents is an almost complete lack of side effects. These drugs can be assigned to different age groups of patients without any limitations and polyvalent bacteriophages can be used to obtain the results of bacteriological research. The possibilities of using bacteriophages in treatment, together with probiotics and synbiotics, have proven their safe use in patients of any age and pregnant women.

The most preferred bacteriophage is the use of polyvalent phage preparations. Pathogens against which it is directed (staphylococci, streptococci, pathogenic enteric bacteria and pseudomonas, proteus, and klebsiella) are the causative agents of severe surgical and intestinal infections, the lethargic level may reach up to 30-50%. However, their use in pyobacteriophage is effective in 70-90% of cases. It is important to emphasize that the use of polyvalent pyobacteriophage does not exclude the use of other anti-inflammatory and antibacterial drugs. The absence of contraindications and complications when using drugs of bacteriophages, allows them to be used in combination with other drugs.

CHAPTER FIVE

Practical Applications of Bacteriophages

The lysis effect of bacteria phages can be used with curative - prophylactic purposes in various diseases as in dysentery, cholera, various purulent-inflammatory diseases, etc. The standard phage, including international ones, are used for phage typing of pathogens of diseases (cholera, typhoid fever, salmonellosis, diphtheria, staphylococcus and other diseases). Typically, such patients are assigned with antibiotics, but due to the fact that constantly mutating bacteria become resistant to antibiotics, their effectiveness is diminished in the recent years. The attention of researchers attracted bacteriophages - viruses, bacteria devour. Unlike antibiotics, which eliminate both harmful and healthy microflora of the organism, bacteriophages are selective in nature.

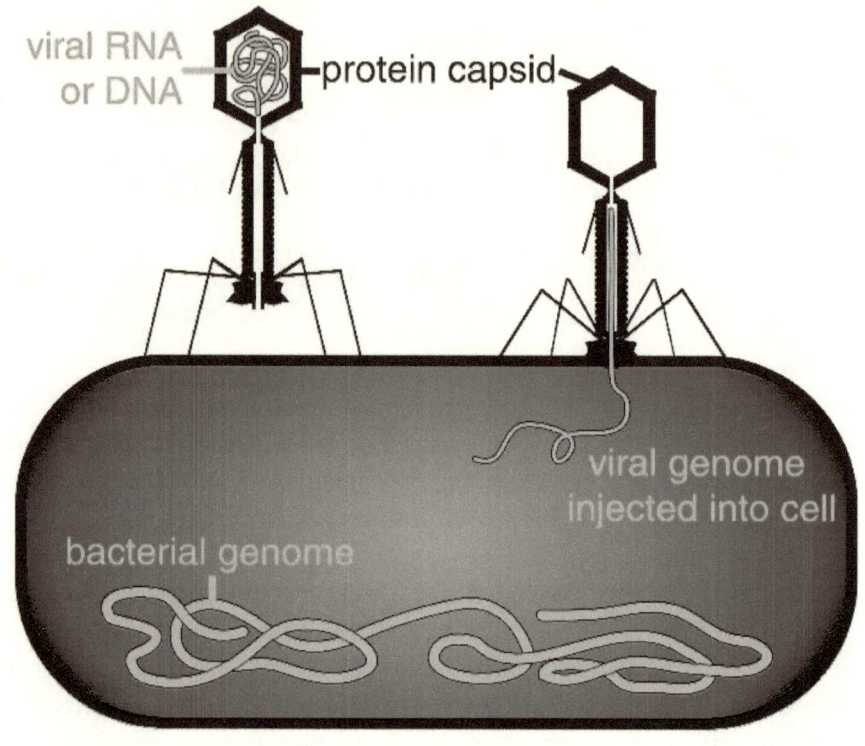

by phage:Adenosine, bacteria + composition: Thomas Splettstoesser (www.scistyle.com) (Eigenes Werk) [CC BY-SA 3.0 (http://creativecommons.org/licenses/by-sa/3.0)], via Wikimedia Commons

How do bacteriophages penetrate the body? They penetrate only in certain cells and interact with the cells' DNA, creating a lysogenic or lytic effect. While lytic types of bacteriophages kill them and allow them to multiply rapidly, lysogenic phage type penetrates into the genome of the bacteria, their synthesis, and the further transition from one generation to another. Information about bacteriophages appeared more than a century ago when they were used to treat staphylococcus. They are now widely used for the prevention and treatment of intestinal, staphylococcus, streptococcus, typhoid and many other infections.

Modern medicine is seeking methods, which do not use live bacteriophages and enzymes acting on pathogenic bacteria by lysing it. Their use may be in the form of a nasal or oral spray, toothpaste, foods, and food supplements. The efficacy of bacteriophages is the absence of contraindications and complications, compatibility with other drugs, and active influence on antibiotic-resistant germs. Because of these properties, bacteriophages are being assessed as future drugs for a successful fight against infections.

The important advantages of phage therapy are: they are highly sensitive to the pathogenic microflora, the possibility of the initial application of small doses of a bacteriophage, compatibility with all kinds of traditional antibiotic therapy, and the absence of contraindications to prophylactic and phage therapy. In nature, microorganisms completely resistant to bacteriophages do not exist. Importantly, the bacteriophage propagation is possible only in the presence of bacteria sensitive to it. After the elimination of the last microbial cell during an outbreak of an infectious type, bacteriophages cease to be active and completely eliminated from the body.

The observed decrease in the therapeutic action of antibiotic drugs used in clinical practice, led to the addition of an alternative to antibiotics. bacteriophage preparations are not in any way lower in antimicrobial efficacy. They stimulate local factors to produce specific and nonspecific immunity and, thus, do not cause toxic and allergic side-effects. Bacteriophages are appointed orally (interior), as well as used for irrigation of wounds, for introduction into the drained cavity - peritoneal, pleural, nasal sinuses, middle ear, abscesses, wounds, uterus, and bladder. In an oral and aerosol application, and when applied to the surface, the Bacteriophages penetrate the mucosal layer, are able to quickly penetrate into the blood and lymph through the kidneys and are then excreted in the urine. As shown in many studies, within 30 min. after administration of bacteriophages, phage particles have been detected in the urine, and their maximum concentration is achieved in the urine, 6-8 hours after ingestion.

CHAPTER SIX

Advantages of Bacteriophage Preparations

The advantages of the bacteriophage preparation's narrow specificity of action is that, unlike antibiotics, it does not cause the inhibition of normal microflora and it has a proven stimulating effect on bifidobacteria. Staphylococcal bacteriophage - a key component of the intestinal micro biocenosis. The use of bacteriophages for treatments of infectious diseases and specific factors stimulating nonspecific immunity, is especially effective in treating chronic inflammatory diseases, in the area of immunosuppressive states in the bacterial carrier.

Experimental work and long-term clinical observations proved the impossibility of the transmission of antibiotic resistant plasmids and toxigenicity to bacteriophages because they are polyclonal complex virulent bacteriophages.

In Russia, the CIS countries, Poland, France and Spain, bacteriophages are widely used in human and veterinary medicine. A wealth of experience in the use of bacteriophages in the treatment of intestinal infections, shows the high clinical efficacy of phage therapy of acute and chronic dysentery, salmonellosis and so on. It has also shown a high epidemiological efficacy for prophylactic use in treating dysentery, typhoid and salmonella. These were from controlled epidemiological experiments on bacteriophages, conducted in preschool institutions and industrial enterprises. The usage of bacteriophages showed good results in the treatment of diseases caused by conditionally pathogenic bacteria, such as dysbacteriosis, purulent skin lesions, internal organs, musculoskeletal system, urogenital system, circulatory system and respiratory systems, including in newborns and infants.

An important condition for ensuring the effectiveness of the treatment of phage preparations is determined by the phage sensitivity of pathogen. Currently, there is a renewed interest in phage therapy in surgery, urology, ophthalmology, traumatology and so on. Therapeutic and prophylactic drugs are composed of polyclonal phage virulent bacteriophages, within a wide range of activities, and active against bacteria resistant to antibiotics. They are produced in the form of liquid, tablets with an acid-resistant coating, suppositories, ointments, and liniments.

The success of active therapeutic - prophylactic agents of bacteriophages against septic and enteric disease are quite high, from 72% to 90%, including against hospital strains, which are characterized by multiple antibiotic resistance. These drugs of bacteriophages undergo constant adaptation to the circulating strains of bacteria by updating phage genes. This feature distinguishes the phages from other antimicrobial drugs - antibiotics or vaccine eubiotics, where production strains, producer strains or synthesized substance is not subject to any modifications. This plasticity of bacteriophage preparations ensures the continuation of the primary phage-resistant pathogens.

Long experience of phage therapy at the institute of urology, showed us a result of the adaptation of the "bio" commercial bacteriophage to hospital strains, which are circulating in the urological clinic. The phage sensitive strains increased by 15% and exhibited level or higher sensitivity to the latest foreign antibiotics. In the area of extended use of bacteriophages in a hospital among hospital strains, phage-resistant formation was not observed, while antibiotic resistance decreased. The clinical efficacy of phage therapy was observed in 92% of cases, often surpassing the results of antibiotic therapy. Because of the absence of contraindications and complications when using bacteriophage drugs, they can be used in combination with other medicines, including antibiotics, are active against antibiotic-resistant strains and are adaptatable to modern pathogens. All this allows us to assess the preparations of bacteriophages as a highly effective and long-term means of emergency treatment of purulent, septic and enteric infections. However, phages may be used not only for treatment but also for prevention of infectious diseases. They can be administered to pregnant women, lactating mothers and children of any age, including premature infants. The basic condition for their successful application is through selected cultural sensitivity to the corresponding phage. There was a surprising pattern: in contrast to antibiotics, the sensitivity of clinical strains of microorganisms to bacteriophages is stable and tends to rise, which can be attributed to the enrichment of medicinal products with the new generation of phages. In addition to medical applications, bacteriophages are widely used in veterinary medicine and are particularly effective in the treatment of staphylococcal bacteriophage mastitis in cows. Bacteriophage preparations can be appointed internally, with diseases of internal organs, or locally, directly applied to a lesion. The action of the phage manifests within 2-4 hours after administration (which is especially important in the intensive care unit). Bacteriophages penetrate into the blood and lymph and are then excreted through the kidneys and urinary tract in the form of urine.

CHAPTER SEVEN

Pros and Cons of Bacteriophages

The narrow range of exposure
Pro:
Used when necessary to eliminate pathogenic bacteria, but preserves the normal flora. In this situation, the use of antibiotics can lead to serious consequences, such as infection of clostridium difficile.
Con:
This limits the possibility of replacing an antibiotic phage therapy capable of influencing a wide range of bacteria. However, this disadvantage may be offset by the use of phage mixtures.
Needless multiplication
Pro:
Phages (as opposed to antibiotics) should not be delivered to the site of infection at a high concentration. Their needless multiplication (which is due to perishing bacteria) leads to a much higher concentration of phages exactly where they are needed.
Con:
Applied dose of phages increased, due to needless multiplication. If a particular phage had some toxic properties, it could be a problem. However - it is very unlikely.
Easy to obtain
Pro:
Phages are numerous and easily isolated from the substrate, in contrast to antibiotics.
Stimulation of bacterial virulence
Con:

Phages, especially moderate, can encode or include bacterial virulence. It is recommended to use virulent phages, i.e. those, which immediately kill those susceptible bacteria and which does not cause lysogens

Easy to produce new phages

Pro:

Phages can be modified in many different ways. Mutagenesis evolution in vitro or in vivo; molecular methods can be used to obtain new phage therapeutic opportunities.

Endotoxin by bacteria

Con:

Simultaneous death of a large number of gram-bacteria leads to the formation of a mass of Endotoxin (LPS). More research is needed to carefully use phages in situations where this may be a problem.

Activity against drug-resistant bacteria

Pro:

Antibiotic resistance and resistance to phages – largely unrelated phenomena.

Immunogenicity

Con:

Using phages can be limited, due to inactivation of their innate and adaptive immune responses. Using other or specially selected phages can solve this problem.

Shelf life is dependent on storage conditions.

Con:

Some phages or phage preparations require storage in a refrigerator.

CHAPTER EIGHT

Uses of Bacteriophages or Phage Therapy

(Samples)
Intestinal diseases
In the digestive tract, trillions of microorganisms arrive on a daily basis, which forms a natural ecosystem, called the intestinal microflora. Every day our body needs to maintain a certain balance of microorganisms. The presence of bacteriophages is a key component of the intestinal mucosa, which plays a crucial role in stabilizing the microbial balance. Bacteriophages are viruses that are everywhere and live in bacteria. They, like other viruses, have their genetic material enclosed in a protein coat. They are divided into groups that have certain characteristics and, within these groups, there are hundreds of different subtypes. Many experts believe that phages can be a good tool in the fight against pathogens and drug-resistant strains of bacteria. Bacteriophages are present when there are bacteria because they depend on them.

Scientists have evidence that bacteriophages in animals and humans kill unwanted bacteria colonies and control the structure of the colonies of friendly microorganisms in the body. A major role for their existence is the mucus layer. It forms in the intestine, an original habitat. It has been suggested that humans and animals have adapted to the specific phages, and this gives them an advantage in the struggle for survival against certain bacteria. It is proven that sometimes phages enter their genetic material into the friendly bacteria without killing them. This allows the bacteria to have a unique advantage to protect against attacks of other types of bacteriophages. Patients with irritable bowel syndrome, Crohn's disease, ulcerative colitis and some other diseases are likely to have serious problems with the intestinal microflora.

Diseases of Respiratory tract

Acute purulent-inflammatory diseases of the upper respiratory tract is one of the most frequent reasons for patients to visit general practitioners and otolaryngologists. The incidence of rhinosinusitis, tonsillitis, and otitis especially increases in the autumn-winter period and are closely associated with an increased incidence of acute respiratory viral infections in children and adults. Diseases of the upper respiratory tract of viral etiology are often accompanied by the activation of conditionally pathogenic microflora and colonization of the respiratory tract by pathogenic bacteria. This leads to the development of purulent diseases of the upper respiratory tract.

Moreover, inflammation may be a bacterial complication of a viral infection, but sometimes bacterial infections can accompany from the beginning. Thus, in children, the importance of etiologic viral and bacterial associations are observed at 25-30% of acute respiratory diseases. This significantly increases the incidence of chronic suppurative rhinosinusitis in recent years. The alleged reasons for this are the changes in the nature of the immune response at the local and systemic levels. To adequately treat and prevent the transition of inflammatory diseases of the upper respiratory tract, one needs to identify the pathogen and employ timely use of effective isotropic drugs with antibacterial activity.

For many decades, chemotherapeutic antibiotics and synthetic drugs with antimicrobial activity have been successfully used for this purpose. However, all of the antibiotics come with the problem of antibiotic resistance to date. New strains of bacteria are formed much faster than the creation of new antibacterial drugs. This contributes to the total use of antibiotics in practice and is not always justified by the appointment of antimicrobial agents by physicians of different specialties. This can be the base of the problem for the development of antibiotic resistance by bacteria.

Moreover, there are economic losses due to the emergence of various forms of antibiotic-resistant bacteria. There are tens and hundreds of millions of dollars spent on it. For example, in EU countries, at least 1.5 billion Euros per year is spent.

The most important roles in the development of bacterial infections of the upper respiratory tract are played by Staphylococcus spp., Streptococcus spp., haemophilus influenzae, moraxella catarrhalisi and number of other pathogenic strains of bacteria. The most serious threat to health, from a clinical and epidemiological point of view, is methicillin-resistance by staphylococcus aureus and pseudomonas aeruginosa.

Over the past decade, the resistance of these bacteria to macrolides and penicillin, which are traditionally and widely used in otolaryngology, has grown significantly. In addition, in recent years, there has been a sharp increase in the number of bacteria that produce β-lactamase extended-spectrum, due to the extensive use of in-patient and out-patient practice of cephalosporins of the first, second and third generation.

In addition, the spread of antibiotic resistance in pathogens of upper respiratory tract disease is a particular problem and raising the incidence of allergic reactions to the administration of antibacterial agents.

Therefore, to date, of special importance is the use of a complementary and effective means of low allergenic potential, allowing the destruction of multi-resistant bacteria. One promising solution to this problem is to expand the use of bacteriophages. Bacteriophages are viruses, which can eliminate bacteria. In the presence of sensitivity to them, are many the bacterial strains; they penetrate into the bacteria, multiply and eventually destroy them. After lysis of the bacteria, phage particles are again ready for action. Phages are specific; unlike antibiotics, they cause the death of only a certain species of bacteria, without inhibiting the patient's normal microflora. Phage pharmacokinetics studies carried out on laboratory animals indicate that phages, with any method of administration, enter the bloodstream, where they are rapidly adsorbed by various tissues. Most often they are found in lymph nodes, spleen, liver, and kidneys.

Since the presence of microbes in the body of the corresponding phages actively proliferate, the duration of their stay in the body increases and depends on the presence of phage sensitive pathogen infection, which can occur even while increasing the titer of the bacteriophage. The average length of stay of bacteriophages in the human body is about 5-6 days. Sometimes this term is increased or decreased.

The range of methods for use of therapeutic phages are very wide. The methods include not only the application to the site of the lesion, but also oral, subcutaneous, intramuscular, rectal and intraperitoneal routes of administration; as well as the effective use of drugs in the form of aerosols and enemas.

The difference between antibiotics and Bacteriophages:

Phages, as well as all other microorganisms, are capable of changing their properties, shape and size of the colonies. They have the ability to be adsorbed on the microbial cell, the spectrum of lytic effect, and show resistance to external influences.

In turn, the bacteria may acquire resistance to individual phages. However, to date, due to the low prevalence of bacteriophage therapy, this problem is not as acute as in the case of conventional antibacterial agents.

According to modern concepts, antibiotics should not be used for the prevention of chronic inflammatory diseases of ENT organs. This is due to their low efficiency in solving this problem, an increased risk of development of antibiotic-resistant strains, and the potential toxicity to the body.

By contrast, the use of bacteriophages as a prophylactic measure has been used for a long time and has proved its effectiveness and harmlessness. For example, the bacteriophages can be used to eradicate carriage of group-A streptococci, without affecting the normal flora of the mucous membranes; particularly the relevant prophylactic use of bacteriophages in the cold season for children who frequently ill, as well as in patients with immunodeficiency of various types.

With the purpose of treatment of bacterial diseases of upper respiratory tract, bacteriophages can be used as an alternative to antibiotics, especially in cases of selection of antibiotic-resistant strains of bacteria, or if the patient has a polyvalent allergy.

A good therapeutic effect is given by bacteriophages and with a joint association with the traditional antibiotic therapy, this approach is justified and has proven clinically effective.

Proper selection and use of bacteriophages are comparable in efficacy to broad-spectrum antibiotics. Moreover, non-toxic phages cause practically no allergic reactions and have no contraindications for use.

Another more important property of phages, is their indirect immunostimulatory effect. It is believed that the destruction of the cell walls of a bacteriophage can act as a kind of vaccine, primarily increasing local immunity. This is especially important in the treatment of frequently relapsing, chronic, suppurative inflammatory diseases of the upper respiratory tract.

The most important condition for ensuring a positive effect phage therapy is to determine the sensitivity of the isolated strain to the bacteriophage preparation being prescribed.

In otolaryngology, various preparations of bacteriophages, used in accordance with the type of agent, are highly effective in the treatment of rhinosinusitis, but can also be used in the treatment of otitis, tonsillitis, and peritonsillar abscess.

At present, the most versatile drug for the treatment of inflammatory diseases of the upper respiratory tract is polyvalent bacteriophage treatment. This solution is for local and external use, as well as for oral administration, which is sterile filtrate phages of Streptococcus spp., Staphylococcus spp., pseudomonas aeruginosa, E-coli, klebsiella pneumoniae, proteus vulgaris, and proteus mirabilis. The complex bacteriophages included in its composition covers almost the entire spectrum of the main causative agents of nosocomial infections. Each component has a sufficiently wide range of action against various bacterial strains.

Accordingly, the phage can affect the sensitivity to anti-bacterial agents, and poly antibiotic resistance of cells to the pathogen. At the same time, phage is able to perform lysis of the pathogen cells, until their complete elimination from the inflammatory focus, without disruption of microbiocenosis.

The use of phages cause little to no allergic reactions and toxic effects as do antibiotics. The absence of adverse side effects makes it more available and effective to use in sensitive patients, as in children of all ages and pregnant women.

In the treatment of chronic suppurative rhinosinusitis, polyvalent bacteriophage is purified to effectively eliminate the pathogenic bacteria from the source of inflammation and stimulates local cellular immunity. This helps to reduce the frequency of relapses of rhinosinusitis in comparison with antibiotic therapy.

The following regimen is recommended for rhinosinusitis to achieve eradication of the causative agent of the inflammatory focus and achieve the best clinical effect:

1. After the maxillary sinus cannulation is rinsed with sterile 0.9% solution of NaCl, introduce into the cavity, through a sinus catheter, 5 ml of purified polyvalent- bacteriophage. The procedure is repeated two times per day for 5-6 days, and then the catheter is removed.

2. Over the next 10-15 days, repeat the installation of purified polyvalent-bacteriophages with 5 drops in each nostril, 3 times a day.

In the complex treatment of external and acute otitis, the application of 2-10 ml of bacteriophages into the ear, 1-3 times a day, is recommended. When tonsillitis, use rinsing solution with bacteriophages, 3 times a day, instead of antibiotic therapy.

Thus, the therapy of inflammatory diseases of ENT organs, with the help of bacteriophage, is approaching a promising direction and should be considered as an alternative to antibiotic therapy or as an adjunct treatment for traditional therapy with antibacterial agents.

Urological diseases

The use of bacteriophage preparations in the treatment of urological diseases. Despite the variety of products offered for the chemotherapy of bacterial diseases (more than 600 items, including more than 100 antibiotics), urinary tract infections, to date, rank first among all hospital infections.

Difficulties treating urinary tract infections are due to many factors. The introduction of endoscopic interventions (both therapeutic and diagnostic in nature) and high-tech in urological practice, despite the positive aspects, has created a number of problems, including a new entrance gate of infection being opened and an increase in the number of operations on elderly and senile patients with weakened immune systems. Persistent drainage, stones, and residual urine are targets for colonization and breeding places of hospital microflora. The predominance of the role of opportunistic pathogens in the development of nosocomial urinary tract infection, led to a decrease in the effectiveness of treatment and created difficulties in the selection of therapeutic drugs, especially for patients suffering from chronic inflammatory diseases of the kidneys and urinary tract. The original, natural, old antibiotic resistance does not disappear and the bacteria are gradually improving the mechanisms of sustainability and developing protective factors against new groups of antibiotics, such as cephalosporin third-generation, or fluoroquinolones.

Antibiotic treatment can cause the development of dysbacteriosis. In the case of the use of antibiotics against the background of established intestinal dysbacteriosis, antibiotic therapy can enhance the degree of its severity. In addition, antibiotics reduce the colonization of the intestinal microflora and thus reduce the immunity, as well as increase the permeability of the intestinal wall, facilitating the penetration of opportunistic pathogens in the blood stream, the internal organs and the development of a secondary site of infection. Good prospects for an antibacterial therapy are bacteriophage preparations.

Therapeutic and prophylactic bacteriophages contain polyclonal virulent bacteriophages' wide range of actions, including being active against bacteria resistant to antibiotics. Phage therapy can be successfully combined with the appointment of antibiotics.

The modern release preparations of bacteriophages against major pathogens of nosocomial infections, such as staphylococcal, streptococcal, klebsiella, proteus, pseudomonas, and so on. The advantage of these drugs is the strict specificity of action, since they only cause the destruction of its particular type of bacteria without affecting the normal intestinal flora of the patient, unlike antibiotics. The usage of bacteriophages showed good results in the treatment of dysbacteriosis, as well as surgical, obstetric, and ENT infections. Domestic neonatologists also reported that there is a high efficiency of the treatment produced by phage therapy for septic infections in young children.

Phage therapy was used mainly in the treatment of chronic infectious and inflammatory urological diseases, as in chronic cystitis, chronic pyelonephritis, chronic prostatitis, urethritis, festering wounds, and in some cases of an acute septic condition of the patient. Phages are applied through drains into the bladder (50 ml, 1-2 times a day), directly into the wound (10-20 ml), or in the kidney pelvis (5.7 ml) and internally, via oral application (100 ml daily dose in a day for 30 minutes before eating). The course of treatment is 7-10 days.

Satisfactory clinical analyses were obtained at 2-4 days of treatment with bacteriophages, showing reduction of the symptoms of intoxication, dysuria, reduced body temperature, and improvement of bowel function (especially in children). General bacteriological efficacy was over 84%, clinical - over 92%. The clinical efficacy of phage therapy is almost comparable to that of the group of patients who were treated with modern antibiotics - fluoroquinolones.

Thus, the bacteriophage of urinary tract infections is effective for independent treatment or can be used in combination with antibacterial chemotherapy.

As a harmless biological treatment, bacteriophage can be used in young children. For positive results when using bacteriophages, it is necessary to conduct a preliminary study of sensitivity to its microorganisms. When using bacteriophages in large hospitals, it is appropriate to include in the production strains, which are prepared for commercial drugs, hospital strains of chronic inflammatory diseases, specific to the hospital. The domestic bacteriophage preparations are relatively cheap, which is of great economic importance in the treatment of patients with urinary tract infection.

CHAPTER NINE

Phage Therapy an Alternative to Antibiotics

Many experts believe that phage therapy in the near future will produce a revolution in the fight against infections.

The familiar and common antibiotics that healed billions of people in the twentieth century today are becoming less effective. Famous bacteriologists have long predicted the emergence of a critical situation in medicine. Moreover, it is a complex situation, not always justified by prescribing physicians, the free sale of pharmacy, self-medication and widespread use of antibiotics in animal husbandry.

According to the latest results of the WHO study, most microorganisms known to humanity in 10-20 years will acquire resistance to antibiotics. Therefore, new methods are simply necessary to further cope with illnesses. As immunologists argue, the use of bacteriophages will be a panacea for disease.

The introduction of new strains of bacteria is much faster than pharmacologists produce new antibiotics. Therefore, antibiotic-resistant microorganisms are more abundant than antibiotics, which allows them to win; all because of the expensive production process, which is not always justified. Therefore, today it is very important to use additional and highly effective drugs, which are bacteriophages.

Phages are especially indispensable in the fight against nosocomial infections. The fact is, in medical institutions, organisms being transferred from person to person can mutate and develop resistance to antibiotics. However, phages are always ready to come to grips with pathogenic microorganisms and are able to evolve along with them. Therefore, no new antibiotics need to be invented and the existing phages are enough to eradicate bacteria that cause diseases

Bacteriophages are living organisms and that is their main advantage over synthetic drugs. Of course, skeptics will note the slowness of phages as they gradually destroy the pathogen. However, they do not violate the microflora of the human body and do not lead to dysbacteriosis and other diseases. Besides, in the case of serious diseases, phages can be combined with a variety of drugs, including antibiotics. Their advantage lies in the fact that they have an immunostimulating effect, and are useful in preventing infections.

Scientists say that as a result of microbial resistance to antibiotics should be supplemented by treatment with other dosage forms, particularly bacteriophages. In most European countries, these drugs are used safely in the 80s, and as a monotherapy and in combination with antibiotics. Besides bacteriophages used not only for treatment but also for prevention of bacterial infections, septic, intestinal and other diseases.

Pharmaceutical formulation based bacteriophages will be used in the future and can be highly effective in the treatment and prevention of infections. In fact, proteins, the basic building material of viral cells, are nothing more than a new generation of drugs to which pathogens will not be able to acquire resistance. In fact, the potential is for more bacteriophages than antibiotics, but for a number of reasons, they are not widely used in the West. However, to date, molecular biology based on the results obtained in the study of bacteriophages. Recent laboratory research conducted by scientists, has given us the opportunity to study, in detail, not only the structure but also all the stages of interaction between phage and host of pathogenic bacteria. The knowledge gives an opportunity for a fresh look at the possibility of phage use for therapeutic purposes. Scientists say that improvements in the range of existing drugs and production of new drugs has greatly increased the range of diseases against which you want to use bacteriophages. Many pharmacologists believe that antibiotics should be used in cases of very severe illness, but in less severe or chronic forms of various diseases, it is better to give preference to bacteriophages.

In the winter of last year, in the Central House of Scientists, RAMS leading scientists (including microbiologists, epidemiologists, and clinicians) decided that phage therapy is a very promising direction in pharmacology, and should be given immediate attention. In addition, phage therapy has a number of advantages over other drugs because of the precise directional exposure to a particular bacterium, the absence of side effects and complications, the possibility of complex application with probiotics and synbiotics, and safety of application for people of any age, including children and pregnant women. Also, phages do not cause dysbacteriosis and do not violate the intestinal microflora.

Different levels of resistance to bacteria and viruses to all kinds of antimicrobial agents called "antimicrobial resistance"

The reasons for the rapid adaptation of microorganisms to antibiotics:

- Constant use of antibiotics for self-medication, as well as when they are not effective - especially in respiratory infections, cough, flu, fever, and diarrhea;
- Total use of antibiotics in agriculture for preventing the development of diseases that can be transmitted to humans through food. As a result of such precautions, we regularly consume antibiotics, through our meat and vegetables.
- The ability of bacteria to mutate rapidly and adapt to different antibiotics.
- Avoiding the full course of antibiotics.
- Bacteriophages and antibiotics do not compete with, and act together with them:
- Antibiotics can be compared with the heavy artillery. They should be used when you need urgent intervention, and only if their use is much more important than the side effects that they can cause.
- Full production cycle of bacteriophage is much cheaper than antibiotics.

The main disadvantages of antibiotics:

- The occurrence of allergic reactions, especially in most of the earlier generation antibiotics.
- Some antibiotics can lead to kidney damage and hearing functions.
- Violation of enamel and darkening of teeth in children, due to the fact that tetracycline is accumulated in the bone.
- Taking certain antibiotics leads to the development of anemia.
- Antibacterial adversely affects the intestinal flora and leads to dysbacteriosis.
- Violation of growth and hair loss is also quite common in medication.
- Antibiotics are undoubtedly necessary, but not always.

It sometimes happens that bacterial infection complicates a viral infection and it is believed that the earlier a course of antibiotics is used, the more effective treatment will be. However, it is better to give preference to other drugs. For example, if Staphylococcus aureus is constantly dwelling in the nasal mucosa, it should be treated with an antistaphylococcal bacteriophage. Sensitivity to this staphylococcus bacteriophage can be checked with the help of bacterial culturing in the laboratory. Also, in some cases, effective use of immunoglobulin, for example, staphylococcal toxoid. Antibiotics, in this case, will be ineffective.

CHAPTER TEN

The Resistance of Microorganisms and Ways to Overcome it

Resistance to antibiotics means the ability of a microorganism to carry significantly greater concentrations of the drug than other microorganisms of the same type, or to evolve in such concentrations that exceed the macroorganism achieved in the introduction of antibiotics, as in sulfonamides and nitrofurans in their therapeutic doses.

Resistant strains of microorganisms occur when you change the genome of a bacterial cell, as a result of spontaneous mutation. The latter is not connected with a direct effect on bacterial DNA by antibacterial drugs that act as a selective agent. In the process of selection, the impact of chemotherapeutic compounds on susceptible microorganisms are killed and resistance is stored, multiplied and spread in the environment. Acquired resistance is fixed and inherited by subsequent generations of bacteria.

The rate of development and degree of stability are associated with the appearance of the strain of the pathogen. The fastest and often most resistant to antibiotics occurs in staphylococcus, escherichia, mycoplasma, proteus, and pseudomonas aeruginosa. Among pasteurella, clostridia, group-A streptococci, anthrax and hemophilius resistant strains relatively rare.

The most common genetic basis of resistance in bacteria is the presence of extrachromosomal sustainability factors to drugs - plasmids and transposons.

Bacterial plasmids associated with the transfer of drug resistance markers in the conjugation process cells are called R-factors. Plasmid resistance R (conjugated) is made up of two components - the RTF stability of transfer factor, providing the transmission of genetic information, and the r-factor, responsible for antibiotic resistance. In some cases, r-factors (unconjugated plasmid) in bacterial cells exist independently. Intermicrobe transfer of r-factors can be accomplished by mobilizing them and co-integration with the conjugating plasmid. R-factor can simultaneously contain 1-10 or more determinants of resistance to various antibacterial compounds.

Transposon elements - are the DNA fragments that are free to move from one replicon to another. Transposons define different phenotypic traits of the bacterial cells, particularly antibiotic resistance, and facilitate the transfer of antibiotic resistance determinants between chromosomes, plasmids, and phages. They are not subject to the r-system cells that restrict the transfer of chromosomal markers between unrelated species. Genes belonging to the transposon are surrounded by special nucleotide sequences, which ensure their incorporation into the non-homologous gene. Joining stability determinants of the transposon at a constant current, under the selective pressure of the production of antimicrobial agents on the bacterial population, may result in the formation of hybrid plasmids which determine resistance to new combinations of chemotherapeutic agents.

Transposons can be moved within the same species, as well as transferred into new species and genera of microorganisms. It is found that the transposons 1699 T and 1700 T are present in plasmids unconjugated S. marcescens, initially penetrate into the conjugative plasmid of this type, which moves together with other genera in the family Enterobacteriaceae.

The ability of R-factors, transmitted between cells by conjugation or transduction, explains the rapid spread of their microbial populations. Often, as a result of autonomous replication in a cell, there are tens of copies of plasmids, which contributes to the rapid development of resistance, extra-chromosomally.

In transduction, the determinants of resistance to antimicrobial agents move from one cell to another via bacteriophage, which plays the role of a carrier. Phage DNA is integrated into the bacterial genome and replication, chromosome or disentangling of plasmid capture may be genetic elements responsible for resistance. Phage transduction plays an important role in the spread of drug resistance in gram-positive microorganisms, especially staphylococci and streptococci.

Transfer of plasmids during conjugation is carried out by means of sex pili in establishing contact between the two cells. In the cell donor (R +) is a replicated plasmid DNA, one strand of which penetrates into a recipient cell (R-), where it forms a new plasmid. When integrated into the chromosome of the plasmid, the conjugation can be captured from the chromosome of the genetic material of the plasmid DNA. This may be transmitted resistance determinant localized in the chromosome.

The transfer of genetic information between organisms, by transformation, has value only for laboratory research and is not involved in the spread of drug resistance in a production environment.

At the same time, R-plasmid transfer resistance to the drug substance is the most important mechanism of resistance in a bacterial population, especially in the family Enterobacteriaceae. From the point of view of the epizootic, it is the most dangerous determinant of the stability of the transmission from one species of micro-organisms to another.

The circulation of plasmids from animal to animal, from animal to man and from man to animal contributes to the rapid spread of drug resistance worldwide. The resistant plasmids spread by contact and recontamination of drug-resistant microorganisms of large groups of animals, concentrated in limited areas of livestock. Then, there was a transfer of R-factors, from animals to humans; thus, the number of resistant microflora is several times higher than in those not in contact with the animals.

Most strains of E. coli - bowel commensals, can be easily moved within the human and animal populations, and between them, as evidenced by a similar set of plasmid resistance. The bulk of these strains are resistant to most antibacterial compounds. Nonpathogenic escherichia serve as a constant reservoir of resistance plasmids in which the pathogen enters the body, itself carrying no R-factor, but through conjugation may acquire resistance determinants of the drug.

Use of antimicrobial agents in doses underestimated and increasing intervals between the administration of the drug, leads to the creation of antimicrobial compounds in sub-therapeutic concentrations and, consequently, to the selection of resistant organisms.

Antibiotics intended for causal treatment, in order to increase productivity, led to the animals breeding microflora resistant to therapeutic agents. As a result of extensive use of animal tetracycline antibiotics as a feed additive, most strains of Salmonella and Escherichia have acquired resistance to the drugs in this group.

The resistance of microorganisms to the antimicrobial, in the case of both plasmid and chromosomal localization resistance determinant, may be caused by several mechanisms.

The most common drug resistance is associated with the ability of microorganisms to produce enzymes that inactivate antibiotics. A typical example of this type of stability - the ability of lactamases (penicillinases) bacteria hydrolyzes the lactam ring of penicillins and cephalosporins. As a result, Lactam antibiotics communication loses its specific activity against microorganisms.

Another important mechanism that creates antibiotic resistance, is in violation of the permeability of microbial cells to the antibiotic. Thus, the change in staphylococci and pseudomonas aeruginosa lipid composition of the cell wall, breaks its permeability, respectively, for fusidic acid and chloramphenicol. The appearance of non-specific proteins in the outer membrane of E. coli decreases its sensitivity to antibiotics. The polymyxin resistance of pseudomonas aeruginosa is associated with changes in the outer membrane structure that prevents the penetration of the antibiotic in a microbial cell.

Resistance to tetracycline often is inductive. Upon contact with the antibiotic, microorganisms begins the synthesis of specific proteins, which are mainly localized to the outer membrane and restrict flow into the cell tetracycline. Accordingly, induced proteins disrupt the interaction of the antibiotic with the 30S-ribosomal subunit or, by altering the permeability of the cell membrane, provide free access of tetracycline to the bacterial cell.

A possible mechanism of resistance leads to the synthesis of compounds that activate it and through the help of antibacterial agents. Thus, resistance to sulfonamides and trimethoprim associated with the development of low sensitivity to the action of these drugs.

The wide spread of drug-resistant organisms requires the development of a set of measures restricting the circulation of resistant bacteria among farm animals. Measures to limit the spread of drug-resistant organisms should be directed, first, to prevent the formation of resistant populations, and, secondly, to the suppression of already established populations.

One possible way to overcome the drug resistance of microorganisms is a chemical transformation of the molecules of antimicrobial agents, particularly antibiotics, aimed at creating new drugs active against antibiotic-resistant organisms. By transformation, synthesized semi-synthetic penicillins and cephalosporins are created, which are insensitive to the action-lactamases, including methicillin, oxacillin, cefamandole, cefuroxime, cefsulodin and others.

Virtually any antibiotic molecule can be inactivated in the microbial cell by a particular resistance mechanism, so in a while, after you start using a new drug, note the spread of resistance determinants to this compound in plasmids and transposons. In this regard, each antibiotic's effectiveness begins to diminish, which necessitates the synthesis of new antimicrobial agents.

A promising practice in the fight against drug-resistant organisms, is the use of compounds inhibiting certain mechanisms of resistance in a bacterial cell. The greatest success achieved in this direction is as a result of the non-competitive inhibitors lactamases. The first representative is clavulanic acid, its main feature being the ability to irreversibly inhibit penicillinase gram-positive and gram-negative microorganisms. Drugs in this group of sex pili interacting with microorganisms in this connection, primarily inhibit R+ cells bearing resistance determinants. Phosphoglycolipid, widely used in animal husbandry and poultry and is found in the gastro-intestinal tract of farm animals, significantly reduces the number of antibiotic-resistant microorganisms.

Another approach to solving the problem of exposure to the drug-resistant population of microorganisms, is the use of compounds that ensure the elimination of plasmids of drug-resistant bacteria and acts on determinants of drug resistance. One way leading to the elimination of the bacterial cell plasmids, is the use of DNA-tropic substances. Acriflavine and quinacrine cause the elimination of R-factors of Salmonella, Shigella, and Escherichia.

In addition to the direct impact on R-factors, DNA-tropic compounds by reducing mutations and slows the development of resistance of microorganisms to antimicrobial agents. So, quinacrine and acriflavine suppress the development of antibiotic-resistant strains of bacteria to penicillin, ampicillin, neomycin, streptomycin and rifampicin.

Another way to prevent the spread of plasmids resistance, is the use of compounds that effectively inhibit transport processes determinants of stability in bacterial conjugation. Most intensively this process affects rifampicin, ethidium bromide, caffeine, protamine, neomycin, and nitrofurans. Some of these compounds have relatively low toxicity and may be promising when used in veterinary practice. Thus, the introduction of chickens to furazolidones protamine, inhibits the transfer of plasmids resistance in Escherichia.

Disturbances in the transduction chemotherapeutic agents that suppress the transfer of phage determinants of resistance to the drug substance, can limit the spread of resistant strains. Ethidium bromide and rifampicin suppress the frequency of the R-factor in the transmission of E. coli up to 100 times, which is associated with the suppression of phage adsorption on the surface of the recipient cell. Rokkan and chlorhexidine prevent the appearance and accumulation of kanamycin-resistant microorganisms, by anti-phage action, against transducing phages.

The most promising method for real and limiting appearance and accumulation of resistant bacteria in animals, is by increasing the effectiveness of chemotherapy through the use of combinations of different antimicrobials. Thus, the rapid acquisition-resistant Staphylococcus aureus to novobiocin is avoided because of its use of tetracycline. The use of isoniazid with streptomycin prevents the development of antibiotic-resistant strains of Mycobacterium tuberculosis. Methicillin benzyl-penicillin prevents rapid formation of Fucidin resistance in staphylococci.

In addition to preventing the development of resistance, rationally selected combinations of antimicrobials may impact resistant strains of microorganisms using enzyme suppression, inactivating one of the mixture components.

In conclusion, the microorganism's developed resistance to the drugs, can be eliminated by the use of bacteriophages or phage therapy. In addition, this therapy can be combined with an antimicrobial agent to prevent the use of antibiotics for most infections. The limited use of antibiotics, then reduces the chance of acquiring antibiotic resistance.

www.ingramcontent.com/pod-product-compliance
Lightning Source LLC
Chambersburg PA
CBHW020713180526
45163CB00008B/3072